Juicing for Health

The Complete Guide to Juicing for Good Nutrition

RON KNESS

ISBN-13: 978-1533003669

ISBN-10: 1533003661

Contents

Introduction

It's well documented that many of us need to increase our daily intake of fruit and vegetables. We are the champions of the world when it comes to getting enough of the macronutrients carbs, protein, and fat, but we're sorely lacking when it comes to getting more micronutrients.

While the Centers For Disease Control recommend adults consume about 1 ½ to 2 cups of fruit and 2 to 3 cups of vegetables daily, an analysis of American diets between 2007 and 2010 found that 50% of the population ate less than 1 cup of fruit and less than 1 ½ cups of vegetables.

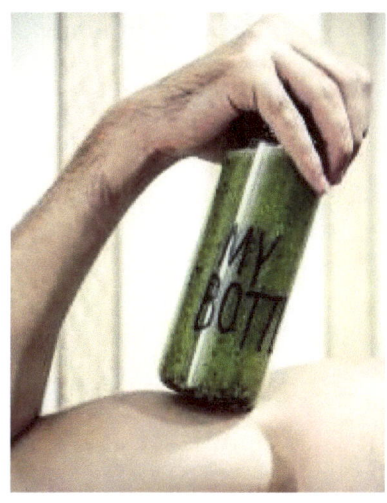

An astounding 76% of people did not eat nearly enough fruit, and 87% did not eat enough vegetables.

Many people simply don't like eating vegetables. Broccoli is tough, cabbage is chewy, and carrots can break your teeth if they haven't been boiled long enough and let's not get started on that stringy asparagus!

However, fruit and vegetables are where essential micronutrients are to be found and juicing is a great way to easily pack more of them into a well-balanced and healthy diet.

Thousands have joined the juicing revolution and for good reason, it is healthy, convenient and allows you to get key vitamins and minerals from plant foods that may be missing from your diet.

General Benefits of Juicing

There are many health benefits derived from juicing. Here are the more popular ones:

- ✓ Increased energy
- ✓ Improved immunity
- ✓ Stronger bones
- ✓ Improved hydration
- ✓ Better skin health and appearance
- ✓ Essential nutrients for general health and to fight chronic disease
- ✓ Weight loss
- ✓ Improve the aging process

Juice Nutrition

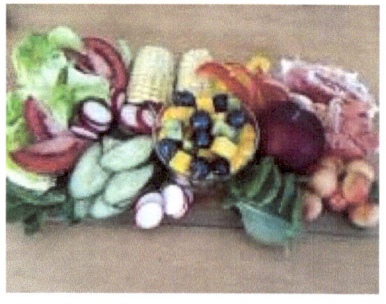

Juicing is a very convenient and easy way to consume more healthy plant foods and the essential nutrients they provide.

Nutrients Exclusive To Vegetables And Fruits

There are micronutrients in produce that you cannot get from any other food. This includes key antioxidants that fight free radicals and protect cells in the body.

Potassium

Potassium promotes proper fluid balance and supports muscle and nerve function. Fresh vegetables are key sources of potassium, including squash, artichokes, carrots, and broccoli.

Vitamin A

Vitamin A supports skin and vision health and also promotes immune system health. Yellow, orange, and dark leafy greens are the best sources, including bell peppers, kale, broccoli, and carrots.

Vitamin C

Vitamin C is a well-rounded antioxidant that enhances the absorption of iron, speeds wound healing and supports immune system health. Citrus fruits, like oranges, lemons, and grapefruits along with broccoli, tomatoes, and green pepper are some of the best sources.

Magnesium

Magnesium supports healthy bones and plays a key role in more than three hundred enzymes in the body.

Folate

Folate is a B-vitamin that plays a key role in the synthesis of red blood cells. Folate is a big part of prenatal vitamins as it prevents birth defects in the growing fetus. Broccoli, tomato juice, and asparagus are your best plant sources of folate.

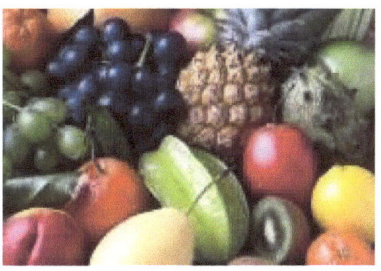

Phytonutrients

According to the National Cancer Institute, phytonutrients may play a key role in preventing cancer and lowering risks for various health problems.

Phytonutrients are active compounds found in plants that protect the plant from pests and other environmental hazards and they do the same for humans.

Three types of phytonutrients

- Organo-sulfurs – mainly found in garlic compounds
- Terpenoids – mainly found in citrus fruits
- Flavonoids - Flavonoids give fruits and vegetables their bright colors, like the red tomato and the purple grape, and the blue blueberry. This group includes the anthocyanins found in blueberries and the quercetin in onions.
- Isoflavonoids and lignans: Broccoli and curly kale are rich sources of lignans, along with cabbage, Brussels sprouts, carrots, and green peppers

Phytochemicals in Fruit

Anthocyanidins found in raspberries, blueberries, blackberries and purple and red grapes help protect from the damaging effects of oxidation.

Phytochemicals in Vegetables - Glucosinolates

According to the National Cancer Institute, cruciferous vegetables, which are part of the brassica family of vegetables, including turnips, rutabaga, watercress, broccoli, kale, cabbage, and bok choy appear to have significant cancer-preventive properties.

Various studies show these vegetables to prevent cancer in different ways:

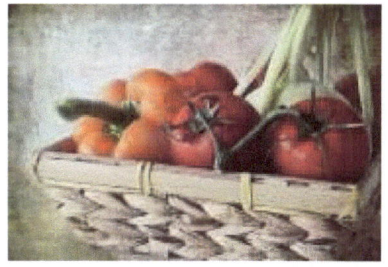

- Protect cells from DNA damage
- Ability to inactivate carcinogens
- Hold antiviral, anti-inflammatory and antibacterial properties
- Induce apoptosis or cell death
- Hinder tumor blood vessel formation and migration, which is required for metastasis

Juicing Can Significantly Increase Intake Of Key Nutrients

If you never get to or don't want to eat whole fruits and vegetables, juicing is a fantastic way of sneaking in some good stuff into your body.

Theoretically, you can get more vitamins and minerals from one glass of juice because you can fit a lot more vegetables into a glass than you can on one single plate, unless you want to chew all day long.

Indeed, you could get your entire daily-recommended amount from just 2 glasses!

Juicing Versus Blending

A common question often asked is *"What is better, juicing or blending?"*

People often ask whether juicing offers more health benefits, or whether blending is the way to go. First of all, let's take a look at the differences between the two.

When you juice fruits and vegetables, you're essentially extracting the water and the nutrients and leaving the pulp behind. Conversely, blenders pulverize the entire fruit and vegetable and instead of making juice, you get what is called a smoothie.

There are many health benefits to both juicing and blending, thanks to all the vitamins, phytonutrients and minerals, you're getting everything you need for a healthier you.

The main difference is that the pulp contains insoluble fiber, which is missing from the juice because the pulp is removed.

Insoluble Fiber

Insoluble fiber is mainly found in whole wheat, brown rice and in the seeds and skins of fruit. It digests slowly and so results in a slower and more sustained release of nutrients.

Health Benefits Of Insoluble Fiber:

- Supports weight loss as it keeps you full longer so you eat less without being hungry

- Supports healthy digestion, and prevents bowel problems

- People often drink a smoothie before a workout to give them a slow and sustained energy drip because the insoluble fiber digests slower than the soluble fiber found in juices

Soluble Fiber

While there is no insoluble fiber in juice, you are still getting a lot of soluble fiber. Soluble fiber attracts water and turns to gel during the digestive process, and causes slower digestion, it is found in apples, blueberries, other fruits and 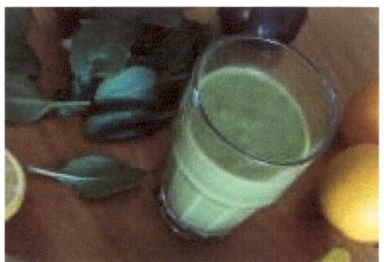 vegetables, beans, nuts, seeds and oat bran, and it is the main ingredient in psyllium fiber supplements.

Soluble fiber absorbs quickly and easily, allowing you to get 100% of key vitamins, minerals, and antioxidants from juiced fruits and vegetables.

Health Benefits Of Soluble Fiber

- Helps keep cholesterol levels healthy and protects the heart.

- Bulks up the stool to support healthy digestion and prevent common ailments, such as diarrhea and constipation and diarrhea. This is why fiber supplements are made mostly from soluble fiber.

- Maintains healthy blood sugar levels to avoid blood sugar spikes that pose a risk for type 2 diabetes and can help those already diagnosed to manage the condition.

- Soluble fiber supports weight loss as it can keep you full longer, while keeping your calorie counts down, especially when its source is fruits and vegetables.

- Older people and those with digestive disorders can benefit from juicing and eliminate the hard to digest insoluble fiber found in juiced or whole fruits and vegetables.

Which Is Better: Juicing or Blending?

The answer is both are great! You don't have to choose because blending complements juicing, and vice versa and either one can help fill the nutritional gaps of the other.

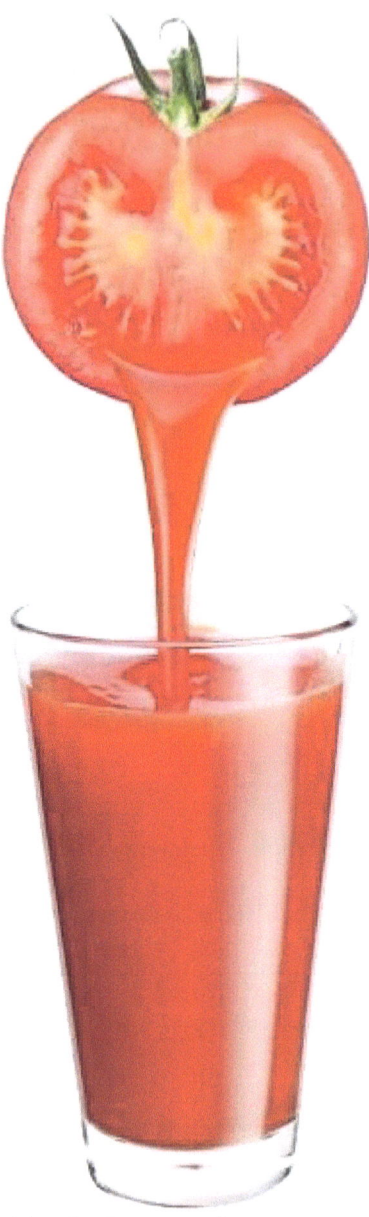

- ✓ Juicing vegetables allows you to get a plethora of key nutrients without the bulk of the insoluble fiber for pure liquid nutrition.

- ✓ Blending and juicing together allows you to make a variety of tasty blends, for example, strawberries don't juice very well, but kale, and spinach does. Therefore, you make your vegetable juice, and then stir in the blended strawberries, and you get the best of both worlds, delicious taste and complete nutrition.

✓ Blending is ideal for the soft produce that cannot be juiced, like avocados, and bananas.

✓ Blending also allows you to get the benefits of the entire fruit, as the fiber content prevents the blood sugar spikes that are seen with high sugar fruit juices.

✓ If you want to boost the nutritional value of your diet, juicing gives you a straight shot of nutrition any time of the day. You don't have to spend all day deciding what fruit or vegetable to eat next - you can get all your nutrients in one go. Excellent!

✓ Juicing allows for an easy way to drink your nutrition, instead of having to chew on a giant plate of vegetables or drinking a thick smoothie. Juicing gives you more choices, due to the great variety of juicable fruits and vegetables.

Taking advantage of both blending and juicing is the smartest way to access the best each has to offer.

Sound nutrition is so important, but so many of us just don't get enough. We are great at getting our macronutrients (protein, carbs, and fat) but we're not so great when it comes to getting enough micronutrients. Juicing and blending is a great way to boost our intake of micronutrients and improve our diets.

The great thing about juices and smoothies is that they allow you to get more fruit and vegetables than you otherwise would.

After all, you can only chew so much kale each day, or peel so many apples.

You get exhausted doing it. You forget to do it.

Juicing and blending makes everything so much easier and so portable.

Juicing Facts and Myths

People who juice are often faced with questions from others who do not understand the benefits of juices. Here are some facts and myths about juicing that you will want to consider:

- **Juice has no fiber in it.** This is a myth. Juice contains plenty of soluble fiber that soaks up glucose and cholesterol, lowering the amounts of these substances in the bloodstream. Soluble fiber also takes on water so the stool is bulked up and bowel movements are easier.

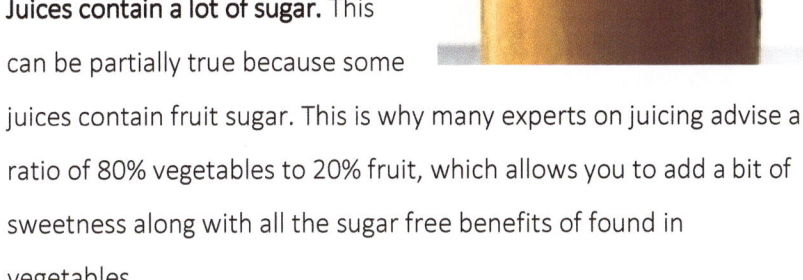

- **Juices contain a lot of sugar.** This can be partially true because some juices contain fruit sugar. This is why many experts on juicing advise a ratio of 80% vegetables to 20% fruit, which allows you to add a bit of sweetness along with all the sugar free benefits of found in vegetables.

- **You can't detoxify on juice.** This is partially true. While vegetables like broccoli, cauliflower, kale, radishes, cabbage, and Brussels sprouts have phytonutrients in them that increase the enzymes in the liver, it is the liver that does the detoxifying. We naturally detoxify ourselves every day, but adding more phytonutrients from juicing to our diets can help.

- **You can kick start a healthy diet or weight loss plan with juicing.** This is absolutely true. Juicing is a great way to detox off junk food, get your body in touch with real nutrition, and kick start your way into a healthy lifestyle.

- **Juicing has no health benefits.** Increasing research studies have shown that drinking vegetable juices will provide you with many health benefits. For example, beet juice can help manage hypertension. There are more and more studies pointing to the health benefits of juicing.

- **Juicing doesn't have protein in it.** You can add many sources of protein to your juice as you are making them. For example, you can add hemp seeds, chia seeds, or a protein powder to the juice for an added boost of protein.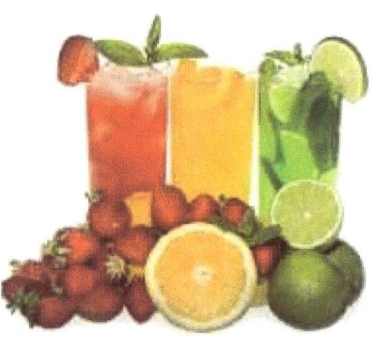

- **Juice diets are just a fad.** This is another myth as juicing has only seen steady growth since the 1980's as people take heed to the lasting health benefits of increasing plant food intake to prevent disease, boost energy and improve overall health and wellness. Carrot juice, for example, has been shown through research to decrease the damage to WBCs in smoking clients.

- **The nutrients leave the juice in the extracted pulp.** This is another myth. When you juice, only the insoluble fiber is removed with the pulp, but many vital micronutrients remain in the juice along with soluble fiber making it a very healthy beverage.

- **It is better to eat fruits and vegetables than it is to juice them.** This is partly true if you are looking for a source of insoluble fiber. The other nutrients in juice can be found whether you eat the vegetable (or fruit) or drink them in juice form. Some vegetables are actually healthier for you in a juice when compared to roasting or otherwise cooking them.

- **Juices can be contaminated with bacteria.** You can get bacteria in juice but it is usually in the manufactured form of juices and not in the juice, you make at home. Wash your hands before you make your juice, peel vegetables before juicing, and wash the vegetables before putting them in the juicer. Drink them right away or store them in the refrigerator for no longer than 72 hours.

- **You can lose your hair if you juice.** This is only true if you have an underlying medical condition, such as hypothyroidism. If you are worried that you might have a condition that leads to hair loss, talk to your doctor before starting a juicing program. Make sure the juice has health-retaining nutrients in it, such as zinc, protein, and biotin.

- **Juicing is much too expensive.** While you do have to invest in a juicer, you should know that it is not much more expensive to juice your vegetables and fruits than it is to eat them whole. If you don't want to waste anything, you can save the pulp for use in soups, cookies, and in other baked goods.

Vegetables: Your Key Players

There is no doubt that vegetables should be the key players in all your juice blends. They have little or no sugar, and offer you only what you need in nutrients that help prevent disease, improve your energy levels, and keep you healthy even into old age.

One of the biggest questions is which vegetables are best for juicing. It's a big question because you have a wide-open field of vegetables to choose from.

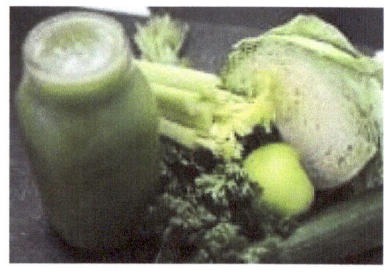

With so much choice, how do you know which will taste better when used in a combination with others, and which offer the best nutritional value?

Your goal is to pick vegetables that produce the biggest yield in terms of taste, the most juice, and the most nutrients:

- Taste - Because without taste, you're not going to want to "brave" juicing ever again and will most likely keep buying those sugar-laden fruit juices from the supermarket.

- Juice - Because without much juice, you're not getting any goodness and the whole exercise is pointless.

- Nutrients - Because it is the nutrients that make you feel GOOD about juicing!

You can juice any vegetable, and vegetables with a high water content, like cucumbers make your base juice, while leafy greens, such as kale and spinach, are what give you so many nutrients.

Best Vegetables For Juicing

Here are some of the top vegetables to put in your juicer, as they are full of quality nutrients and are extremely supportive of good health. Please note that this list is by no means exhaustive and really most all vegetables can be juiced, though not all will yield the same amount of juice. Whichever vegetables you choose, keep in mind that juicing is pretty much a nutrient express train that zooms through your body rapidly. Think of it like a delivery driver who is trying to make record time!

Cucumber

The humble cucumber is one of the hard vegetables that you shouldn't

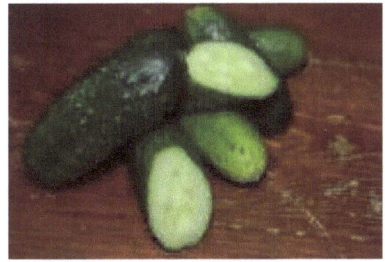

be scared of putting into your juicer. Its high 95% water content makes it a great base juice that offers you excellent hydration benefits.

However, cucumbers also have many health benefits, including potassium, which reduces your risk of stroke, and an anti-inflammatory flavonol that plays a role in brain health along with polyphenols called lignans that may reduce risks for cancer.

They also have plenty of antioxidants such as vitamin C and beta-carotene that fight free radicals.

Cucumbers also promote skin health to make aging easier on the eyes.

Carrots

Carrots add some color to your juice, but there is much more to them as they taste great, compliment all your other vegetables and they are bursting with nutrients.

They contain plenty of vitamins, including vitamin A, vitamin C, vitamin K, and Vitamin B8, and numerous minerals such as potassium, copper, iron, and manganese. As such, carrots can prevent heart disease, lower your blood pressure, and give your immune system a timely boost.

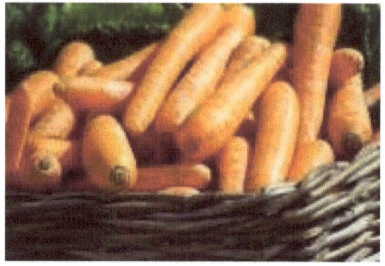

The beta-carotene in carrots, which is responsible for their orange color, is an antioxidant that helps maintain healthy skin and plays a key role in eye health.

Broccoli

Broccoli is considered by kids everywhere and likely some adults to be a really boring vegetable, but broccoli is really supportive of human health and nutrition.

Athletes, bodybuilders, and health nuts include this cruciferous vegetable in their diet to prevent certain cancers, reduce cholesterol, strengthen bones, and help keep their bodies nice and toned. It is high in vitamin K and vitamin E, an antioxidant that protects cells from free radicals, as well as B vitamins AND vitamin C that boosts immunity.

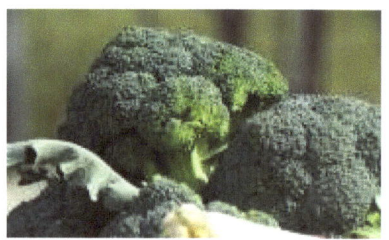

Broccoli juices great and blends well with apples, pears, and even berries.

Sweet Potatoes

For your juice to be the coolest in town, it needs a pinch of sweetness. The best way to get said sweetness is via the smoothest vegetable of them all, the suave sweet potato.

The sweet potato looks the part and tastes the part (and is indeed one of the tastiest vegetables known to man), but it also comes with lots of nutritional value, too.

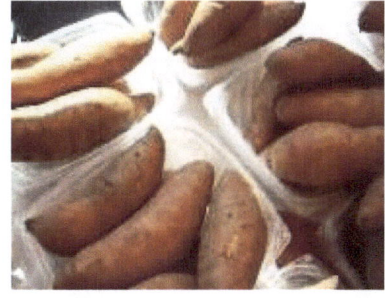

It's rich in vitamin A, vitamin B6 and vitamin C, contains lots of iron and magnesium, and because their natural sugars are released slowly into your blood stream, you don't get any of those nasty spikes in your blood sugar levels.

Cabbage

Cabbage is another great base juice as it is 95% water. If you are like most people, you probably don't like eating cabbage whole. It's big, it's chewy, and it just doesn't go down too well. When you juice it, though, it's pretty amazing.

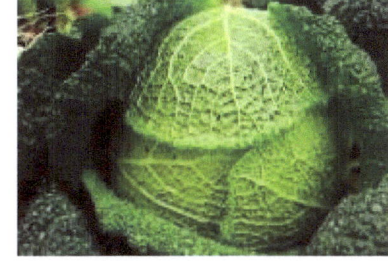

You can actually juice cabbage on its own, though its flavor is much enhanced by apples or carrots. Cabbage juice helps you to lose weight by purifying your intestine so that disposing of waste becomes so much easier. It can also protect you from certain cancers, ward off cataracts, and strengthen your immune system.

Celery

Ah, celery, the slimmest, tallest, and leanest vegetable on the planet. Celery is certainly a great juicing vegetable that's 95% water content allows you to get lots of fresh, nutrient rich juice.

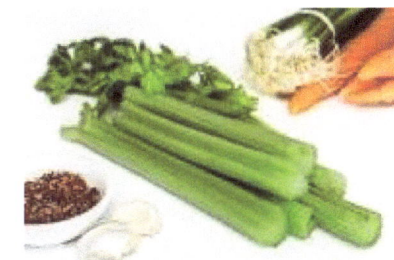

Despite its slim stature, a single stick of celery contains high amounts of vitamin K, vitamin A, vitamin C, folate, and potassium. Make sure to juice the green leaves as they have the most potassium content.

Celery juice blends well with all other vegetables and many fruits and is very refreshing over ice.

Kale

Kale is a powerhouse of nutrition that contains the highest vegetable source of vitamin K, which supports bone health along with calcium, minerals, copper, potassium, iron, manganese, and tons of vitamins.

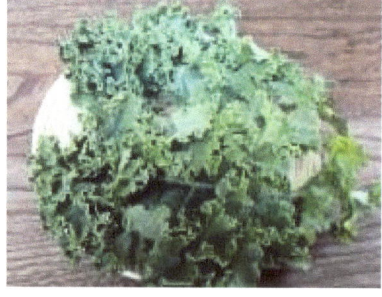

Kale is another member of the cruciferous family, alongside broccoli, and both are noted by the National Cancer Institute as playing a potentially key role in cancer prevention studies.

Low in calories, kale juices great and blends well with many fruits and vegetables. Kale is usually the star of the famous "green juice" that has taken the health world by storm.

Swiss Chard

Swiss chard is another nutritional powerhouse that is high in vitamin K, which assists with blood clotting, and protects your bones.

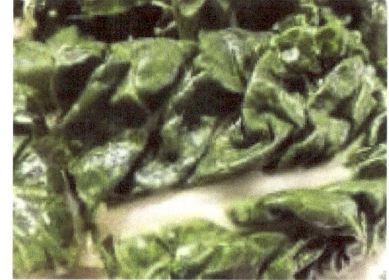

Moreover, you get vitamins A and C, magnesium, potassium, and iron.

If you hate eating greens, juice your chard to get all the health benefits, and it blends great with lemons, ginger, apples, or pears.

Spinach

We all saw Popeye's muscles bulge when he ate his spinach, and yet many of us never touch the stuff. If you hate eating spinach, try juicing it instead.

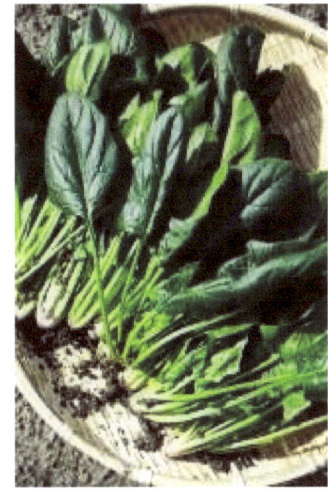

It is an excellent source of vitamins A, C, and E, along with calcium, iron, potassium, protein, and choline that supports healthy brain function.

It blends great with ginger, apples and carrots, and many other gems in the produce aisle.

Kohlrabi

Kohlrabi is a member of the Brassica family that also features cabbage, collard greens, and Brussels sprouts.

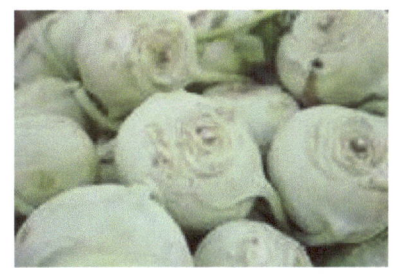

It has a mild sweet flavor and is very low in calories. It gives you lots of vitamin C for healthy immunity, and protects from chronic disease and cancer as it scavenges harmful free radicals that can roam inside the human body.

According to the National Cancer Institute, the phytochemicals in Kohlrabi, including isothiocyanates and sulforaphane may protect from prostate and colon cancers.

It is also rich in B vitamins such as niacin that helps protect the heart, along with the minerals, which include potassium, manganese, copper, calcium, iron, and phosphorus.

The green tops, like turnip greens hold key nutrients so should be juiced for the B vitamins, carotenes, vitamin-A, vitamin K, and minerals.

Juice kohlrabi with kale, carrots, apples, ginger, and lemon, which are all great complementary flavors to its lightly sweet, refreshing taste.

Wheatgrass

Wheatgrass is one of nature's best plant foods. There is a lot of talk that

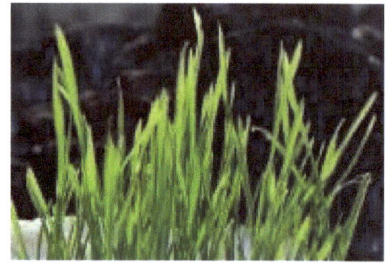

wheatgrass can cure disease, prevent disease and is often over-hyped by the unregulated supplement industry as a miracle cure. Experts, like Mayo Clinic and WebMd advise that there is no scientific evidence to that effect. However, wheatgrass does provide a highly concentrated amount of a wide range of important nutrients that boost your health.

Wheatgrass is the young grass of the wheat plant that contains high amounts of chlorophyll, amino acids, calcium, enzymes, vitamins A, C, E, K, B6, riboflavin, thiamin, 92 minerals, iron, zinc, copper, manganese, and selenium.

Four grams of wheatgrass also contains 252mg or 1260% of the daily-recommended value of Niacin. Niacin or vitamin B3 is important for general good health. It is used in medicine as a treatment to improve high cholesterol levels and reduce risks for cardiovascular disease.

According to WebMD, good evidence exists that niacin helps reduce atherosclerosis, or hardening of the heart arteries.

Wheatgrass must be drank within 15 minutes of juicing to get all its nutritional benefits. It's best undiluted and drank on an empty stomach, (as is true for most fresh juice) in order for the body to absorb all its nutrients.

The Best Fruits for Juicing

Okay, so you've got all your vegetables sorted. You have your cucumber, your spinach, your kale, your sweet potato, and it all sounds great, but what about your fruits?

Fruits are an important part of your juice, not just for the taste and color it adds, but also for the nutritional value.

Apples

Rich in antioxidants that fight the nasty toxins that swim around our bloodstream, apples give your health a boost in numerous ways. They can make your teeth whiter, help you to guard against Alzheimer's, prevent certain cancers, and reduce your risk of diabetes and lower cholesterol.

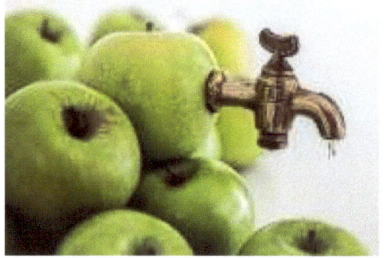

They're an amazing fruit that should really be an essential ingredient in your juices. They are also on the list of the lower sugar content fruit, and especially the green varieties, like Granny Smiths.

Pineapples

Pineapples add fantastic tropical flavor to your juice blends and can help mask the flavor of vegetables for those who just can't stand the taste. This can be especially useful when you are trying to get kids to get their vegetables nutrients.

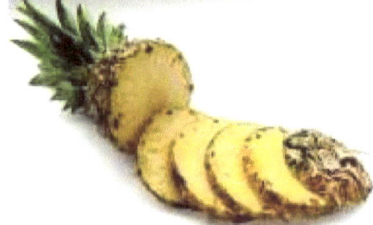

They look amazing and they taste even better.

While pineapples are high in sugar, they are very beneficial to your health. They contain numerous anti-inflammatory, antibacterial, and antiviral properties, which ensure that they can cure skin ailments, prevent hair loss, strengthen your gums and bones, and they can even reduce your risk of developing certain cancers. Keep in mind that pineapples are high in sugar and should be used in moderation.

Tomatoes

Many people still get confused as to whether the tomato is a fruit or a vegetable. Tomatoes are fruits and they taste fabulous. Juicing is a great way to get more of these delicious red lovelies into your diet.

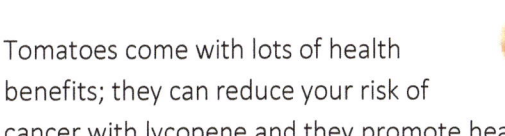

Tomatoes come with lots of health benefits; they can reduce your risk of

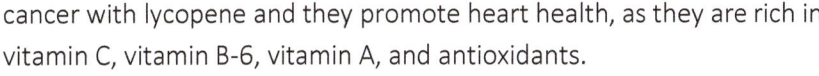

cancer with lycopene and they promote heart health, as they are rich in vitamin C, vitamin B-6, vitamin A, and antioxidants.

They also blend well with your other fruit and vegetables, which ensure a great tasting juice. Fresh tomato juice is refreshing, and can satisfy your sweet tooth in a healthy way when you choose sweet tomatoes like Romano, grape tomatoes or the orange varieties.

Papaya

If you ever get bored of juicing pineapples, you could try papaya. They offer all the lush taste of the tropics that pineapples do, but they have much less sugar and a unique flavor.

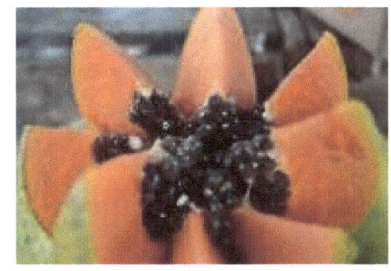

They're nutritional powerhouses with B vitamins, vitamin C, Panthothenic acid, folate, plenty of flavonoids and much much more.

Papaya's lower cholesterol helps with weight loss, boosts immunity, and they are also great for your eyes. Try them!

Berries

Berries are probably the easiest, smallest fruit you will ever juice. They're super convenient, super tasty, and they're absolutely crammed with goodness that contributes to a healthier you.

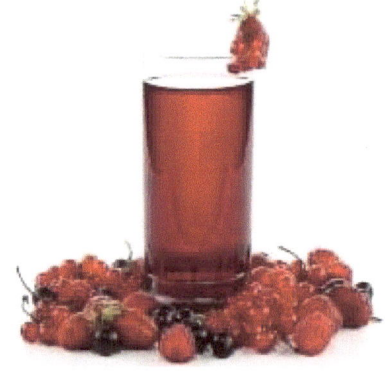

Berries are rich in essential antioxidants to protect cells from free radical damage and they are low in sugar. Perhaps you prefer blackberries today and tomorrow you want to make a strawberry-based juice. Or how about blueberries or raspberries instead? The choice is yours.

Berries do not always juice as well as other fruit, however you can blend them and stir into your vegetable juices, and this also helps to retain their insoluble fiber. Raspberries and blackberries are your lowest sugar options, and blueberries and strawberries have a low to medium sugar content.

Lemons and Limes

You really can't go wrong with lemons. They add a citrus zing to your juice like no other fruit, as they can contribute a fresh, crisp fruity flavor to many different juice recipes.

They're also a miracle cure, as lemons have been known to help with internal bleeding, sore throats, indigestion, dental issues, respiratory disorders, high blood pressure and more.

Lemon juice in particular is super healthy, and can lower your risk of stroke, lower your body temperature if you're feeling feverish and the high vitamin C content in lemons protects your immunity and keeps that cold away.

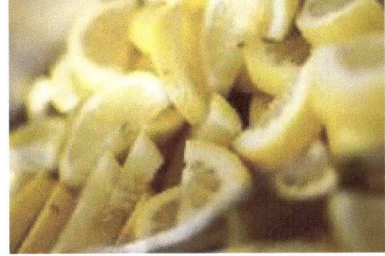

Because many of us simply can't find ways to add lemons to our diet, juicing is the way to go. Lemons have a low sugar content and are ideal for those concerned with high sugar fruit and diabetes. Limes are also great for flavor.

Cherries

Cherries have antibacterial, antioxidant, anti-cancer, and anti-inflammatory properties. The Ellagic Acid in cherries helps protect against cancer and the high iron count supports healthy blood. They are also high in vitamins A and C, biotin and potassium.

Cherries are high in sugar so consider this when choosing them for your juice.

Grapefruits

Grapefruits are loaded with immunity boosting vitamin C and limonene that may help women protect against breast cancer.

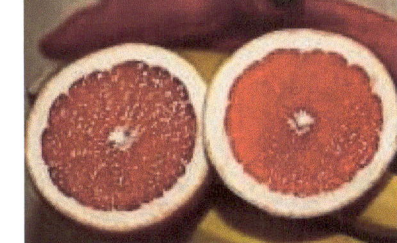

The soluble fiber they contain helps lower cholesterol and they add a fresh zing of fruity flavor to your vegetable juice without too much sugar.

Pink grapefruits are especially tasty.

Avoiding the Sugar Trap

Fruits contain much more sugar than vegetables and some fruits contain much more than others do. Some fruits are very high in sugar, a count that gets even higher when the fruit is juiced, so that fact can negate any benefits they might have. In fact, sugar content is key when considering fruits in your new juicing lifestyle.

Some have so much sugar that you might want to use them in moderation or avoid them altogether, especially if you don't want a spike in your blood sugar levels if you have diabetes or weight issues, and definitely if you are juicing for weight loss.

Experts always tell us to eat more fruit and vegetables. What they don't really go into detail on is the fact that some fruits can actually be harmful when consumed in excess.

This is where juicing can become a problem.

Consider the fact that in order to get about 2 ounces of orange juice, you need to juice 2 medium oranges, so for a regular 6-ounce glass of juice, that is 3 oranges.

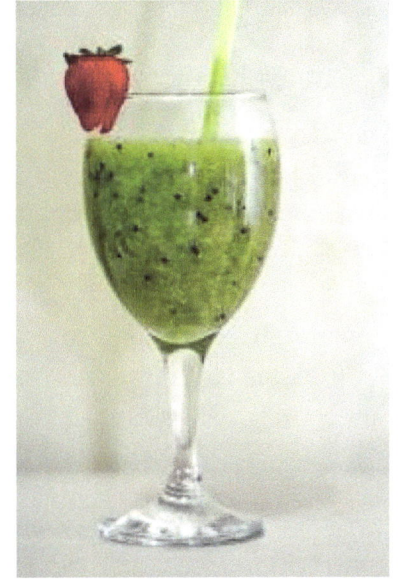

One medium orange has 12 grams of sugar and 62 calories, so when you drink that 6-ounce juice you just ingested 36 grams of sugar and 186 calories just from one drink!

Now, consider if you have or ever will eat 3 oranges in one sitting? You likely would not, so the point is that when you are juicing fruit, you can easily send your sugar and calorie intake through the roof.

Moreover, this is one of the pitfalls to watch out for when starting your juicing journey. People love the sweet taste of fruit juice, and because it's juicing they automatically assume that it's all healthy, but when you look at the sugar and calorie intake, you can 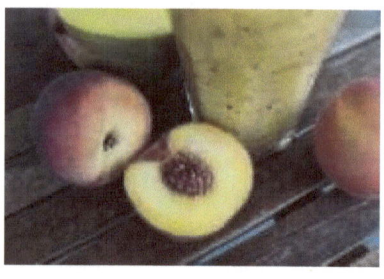 see how quickly this healthy habit can turn ugly for those who drink that 6-ounce orange juice, 2, 3 or 4 times a day!

By the way, US federal dietary guidelines recommend that adults eat 1 1/2 to 2 cups of fruit daily, which is about 2 oranges.

While the sugar from fruit is better for you than table sugar because you are also getting the nutrients that fruit has to offer and not just empty calories as the cupcake does, in excess it can it can harm you just as that cupcake can by contributing to weight gain and increasing risks for type 2 diabetes.

If You Only Juice Fruits, You're Really Missing The Point Of Juicing

If You Mostly Juice Fruits, You Are Missing The Point Of Juicing

The fruit should always be used in moderation to complement and enhance the flavor of vegetables that are the star ingredients in all your juice blends.

Very High Sugar Fruits

Bananas - You see athletes eating bananas all the time. This is thanks to their potassium content, which gives them a boost of energy and also ensures they are easily digested. However, bananas come with a trade-off; containing 14 grams of sugar.

Mango - Mango juice should really be a sweet treat that you have now and then. Just a single mango contains a whopping 31 grams of sugar.

Grapes - Grapes make wine, and wine is sugary. A cup of grapes has 15 grams of sugar. Strangely enough, grapes can also reduce the risk of diabetes and heart disease because they contain resveratrol, a nutrient found in studies to decrease risks for chronic disease.

Figs – One large fig has 10 grams of sugar.

Pomegranate - Pomegranates should be used in moderation as just one pomegranate has 40 grams of sugar. Rather than juice it, you might just want to sprinkle its seeds on your yogurt.

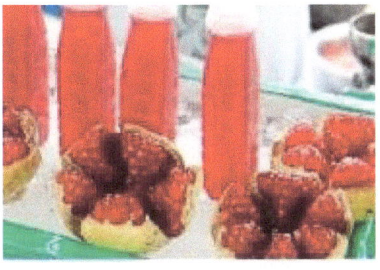

Cherries - Cherries have plenty of health benefits, and they contain many important micronutrients. Unfortunately, a 100-gram serving also contains 13 grams of sugar.

Tangerines – One large tangerine has a whopping 13 grams of sugar.

Fruits Fairly High In Sugar

- Oranges
- Kiwifruit

- Plums

- Pears

- Pineapple

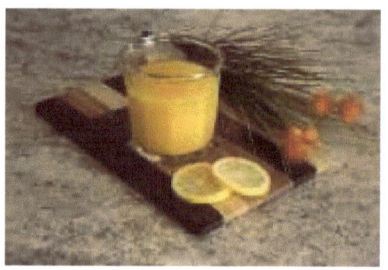

Low To Medium Sugar Fruit

- Blueberries

- Cantaloupes

- Watermelons

- Nectarines

- Papaya

- Peaches

- Strawberries

- Apples

- Grapefruit

- Honeydew Melons

- Guavas

- Apricots

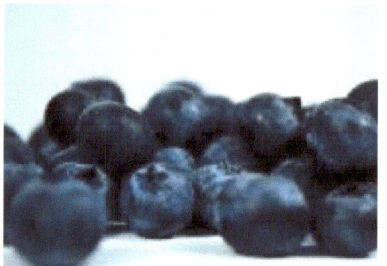

Lowest Sugar Fruit

- Limes

- Lemons

- Rhubarb

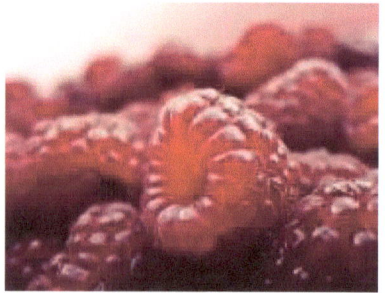

- Raspberries
- Blackberries

Lowering Sugar Intake From Juicing

Many people have no problem juicing fruit and vegetables together. That's the whole point of juicing, to increase your vegetable nutrient intake, right? However, there are a few things to consider.

If you're buying a juicer to make lots and lots of fruit juice because you've been told that it's really healthy for you, it's not. Too much fruit juice with too few vegetables can actually increase your risk of type-2 diabetes, cause weight gain and a whole host of health problems.

Best Practice → Juice mostly vegetables, and a little bit of fruit to add taste

If you're thinking of juicing to lose weight, it is even more important to moderate the fruit intake. Natural sugars, like refined sugars are stored in the body as energy to use for later and when later never comes, it invariably turns these empty calories into fat. They don't get used.

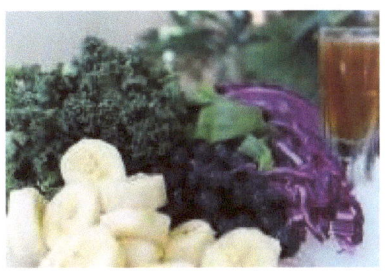

This is why exercise is important so that you do use those sugar calories and burn them off, this way you get all the goodness from juicing, and you get to use all those extra calories as energy, too.

One way to minimize the damage fruit sugar can do is by ingesting as much fiber as you can from the fruit by blending it instead of juicing it.

Sugar is made up of two elements:

- Glucose

- Fructose

Glucose is the good twin; it exists in every single living cell in our body and is a vital part of life. Fructose is the bad twin; once there is too much of it inside your system, it can wreak havoc with your liver.

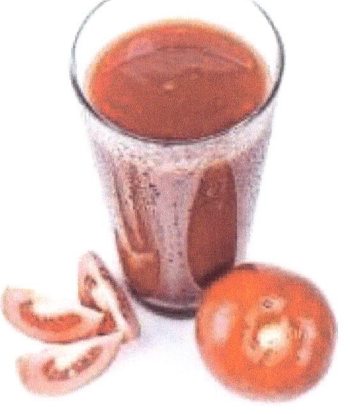

Unfortunately, fruit sugar is mostly fructose.

The problem gets worse when your juice is crammed with sugar, because when that juice sugar enters your body, it races into your bloodstream, which can then cause a nasty spike in your blood sugar levels.

Green Juice 101

Green juice is all the rage and you've probably seen green juice on the shelves at your local supermarket, and at juice bars. It's healthy, tasty, and oh so good.

Green juice is a big deal in juicing, and once you've overcome the strange aesthetic, you'll see how this should be an important part of your juicing lifestyle.

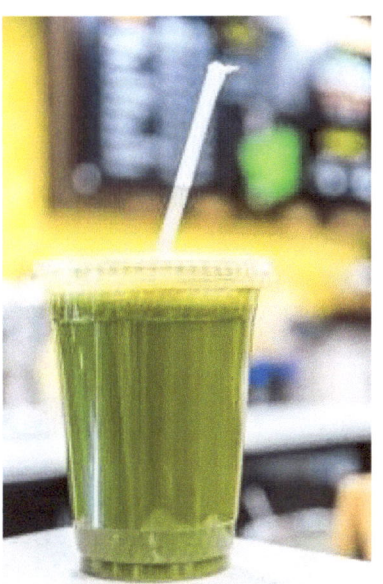

What Is Green Juice

Green juice is a juice that is mostly comprised of dark leafy greens, such as kale and spinach. However, you can also include celery, cabbage, broccoli, and apples. You can also add other flavors, like limes and lemons.

Green vegetables make up the core element of your green juice. Fruits can be added to enhance the taste, but it's the green vegetables that are the star players.

This is where the goodness lies, though, lime juice, mint and ginger root makes it that much better and without detracting from the purpose.

But why should you drink this stuff?

Nutrition

There is a great quote by the Buddha: "To keep the body in good health is a duty. Otherwise, we shall not be able to keep our mind strong and clear."

When you eat the wrong stuff (such as junk food) and drink the wrong stuff (such as soda and too much liquor), your mind is not clear enough to make the right decisions in life. You get brain fog. The fats from junk food don't just get stored in your belly; some of them sneak off and make their way to your brain.

Green juice is absolutely stuffed with top nutrients that give your physical and mental wellbeing a turbocharge. You feel better right away for drinking it and you won't feel like passing out on the couch like after that greasy burger lunch, but will feel energized and clean.

Over time, your skin will glow, the bags under your eyes will disappear, and you'll be more alert and attentive than ever before.

Increase Vegetable Intake

Many can't stand eating green vegetables, but juicing them is much easier to take, and for many people this becomes the best way to boost their nutrient intake from these key plant foods.

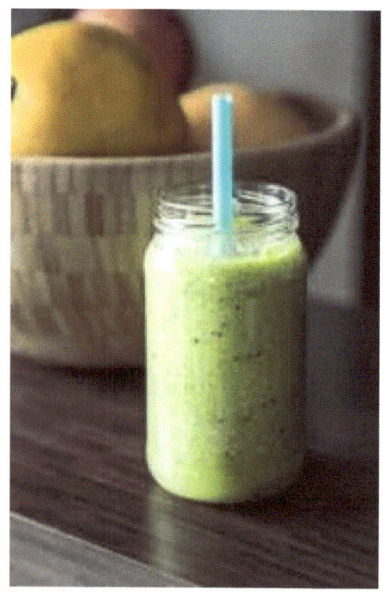

Green juice is great because your body absorbs it very fast. When you eat whole kale, spinach, cabbage and so on, it takes your body a rather long time to process all its nutrients as it takes your digestive system a while to break it down.

When you drink green juice, you're getting all the good stuff straight away, AND you're giving your digestive tract a well-earned break. It's a win-win situation.

You don't feel as full, but you're still energized enough to stay active through the day.

Green Juice Fast

Many use a green juice fast to kick start a weight loss plan, or to detox from junk food and begin a road to healthier eating. Once green juicing becomes a habit, the idea of a mini-fast suddenly seems exciting.

Green juicing is a remarkably clean diet, and if you feel as though your body could really benefit from a detox, there is no better way to do it than via a green juice detox.

Restore Alkalinity

We all have a pH level. It determines how acidic or alkaline our body is. To be really healthy, your pH level has to be in a certain range. If it isn't, it means that you've been getting either too much acid or alkaline from your diet. Drink more green juice to restore pH balance.

Juicing for Weight Loss

Many use juicing to lose weight, but in order to get the best results, it is important to do it right. Here are ten key considerations when juicing for weight loss:

1. **Choose organic:** Use only organic vegetables to avoid toxins, and to increase the nutritional value of your produce and healthy enzyme intake.

2. **Stretch your budget:** Buy from local organic farms and in season vegetables and fruits whenever possible, as they are cheaper and certainly fresher, allowing you to get the most from your juicing dollars.

3. **Watch your sugar intake:** Before you push that fruit through your juicer, STOP and consider this. Fruit is very high in sugar, and you can easily go into a calorie and sugar overload with just a couple of glasses a day, negating your weight loss efforts and the whole point of juicing. One example is the 1-cup of spinach that has only 7 calories and no sugar versus a large orange that has 87 calories and 17 grams of sugar. Make your juices primarily from vegetables and add sweetness and flavor with low sugar fruits like berries, lemons, limes and small amounts of green apples. Ginger is also a great way to add flavor with little calories.

4. **Stick with power vegetables:** Kale, spinach, broccoli, cabbage, greens, celery, cucumbers, and tomatoes are some of your key superfoods for juicing.

5. **Stay active and exercise:** Being active and getting regular exercise is important for weight loss as it allows you to build lean muscle mass, boost metabolism and burn more calories.

6. **Research recipes:** There are hundreds of juice recipes online and in books, and you can benefit from these tried and true blends to get the most flavor and satisfaction from your juice.

7. **Watch out for juice fast pitfalls:** According to the University Of Pittsburgh Medical Center, drastic restriction of caloric intake slows metabolism that can actually make it harder to lose weight. Losing weight too quickly on juice fasts that are too low in calories can cause you to lose more water and muscle than fat, and will likely result in regaining the weight you lost or more. Instead, use juicing to increase your intake of energy boosting nutrient rich vegetables, especially if you are a person whose diet lacks them and to detox off junk food.

8. **Add boosters to your juice:** Add ground chia or flax seeds to your juice, they are nutrient powerhouses that fortify your juice heart-healthy omega-3 fatty acids also found in walnuts. Add protein or whey powder when using juice as a meal replacement to make you feel full longer, feed, and promote lean muscle mass and increase intake of lean protein in your diet.

9. **Eat a balanced diet:** As great as juices are for your health, they are no replacement for whole food. Many people new to juicing attempt to substitute too many meals with juice, which does not supply enough calories to keep you fueled throughout the day, or enough fiber or other nutrients to keep you satisfied and healthy. This can lead to fatigue and hunger, which can quickly lead you to abandon your weight loss efforts. Eating a balanced diet also ensures that you meet all your nutrient needs and not go into starvation mode.

Don't fall for juicing hype: Yes, juicing is a great tool for your weight loss arsenal, but it is not a magic pill for weight loss. Learning to eat right and making profound dietary and lifestyle habit changes is key to long-term weight management success.

Juicer Buying Guide

There is more than one type of juicer, so here are some details so you know what you will find when you shop for yours.

There are two main types of juicers:

- Centrifugal juicer (fast juicers)
- Masticating juicer (slow juicers)

Centrifugal Juicers

Centrifugal or fast juicers are the most popular type of juicer. Why do people love centrifugal juicers? Because they're fast! It's their biggest selling point. If you're looking to make a juice fast, then centrifugal juicers are a good option. They speed up the process, and they clean easy too.

In addition, you get a LOT of juice from your fruit and vegetables, especially if you've invested in a good one.

Fast juicers work by using a centrifugal force that draws out the produce's juicy goodness. The spinning motion much like that of a washing machine separates the juice from the pulp.

The produce is forced down a feed tube (you can just dump whole fruits in there, no need for chopping) before they meet a serrated cutting blade that spins at around 12,000 RPM. The shredded pulp goes into a basket, while the juice goes into a separate container.

Pros

- They juice fast so they are ideal for busy people
- Space saving smaller models

- Do not require the pre-cutting of produce so they save time on prep work
- Work great with hard vegetables, like cucumbers

Cons

- Not the best choice for leafy greens as they will extract less juice than masticating juicers
- Lower juice yield
- Oxidization
- Very noisy models

Masticating Juicers

Masticating or slow juicers do not shred produce with blades, but instead use a slow rotating auger to crush produce against a stainless steel mesh screen at only 80 to 100 rpm, creating no oxidation.

With slow juicers, you get a higher yield and slow juicers are particularly good at making green juices because they get the best nutrients out of kale, spinach and so on.

Pros

- Ideal for leafy greens and can juice wheatgrass
- High juice yield
- No oxidation
- Many models can also make nut butters, juice wheatgrass and even make sorbet

Cons

- More prep work due to a smaller feed chute
- More costly than centrifugal models
- Take more time to extract juice, so slower than centrifugal juicers
- Large and bulky so will need more counter space
- Leaves more pulp in the juice, so may require a strainer (depending on your needs, this may be a pro)

Juicer Shopping Considerations

Juicers Do Not Come Cheap

Juicers are not cheap, so when you consider your purchase, think about this, is juicing just going to be a luxury in your life, or is it going to become a crucial, even necessary part of your new lifestyle? Will you juice ever day or every month?

If juicing is going to be a fundamental part of your life, then it is smart to invest in the best juicer you can afford. If, however, you're only going to be juicing every now and then, then consider a less expensive model that will do the job.

Easy to Use and Clean

This maybe one of your most important considerations because if you have a busy life, spending 20 minutes chopping and prepping ingredients and another 15 minutes on cleaning will be a hassle. In this case, choose a juicer with a big feed chute, the bigger, and the better, as this will require little or no chopping of produce.

There Are Powerful Juicers ... And There Are REALLY Powerful Juicers

There are the really colossal juicers and there are smaller juicers. The bigger models will be very big and powerful, and may be not ideal for novices or even younger family members like teenagers.

If you're just starting out in juicing, consider this in your shopping. If you have a large household, you may want a much larger model that can make more juice for lots of people, versus a one or two person household where a smaller model is idea.

You should also bear in mind that the bigger the juicer is, the harder it's going to be to clean.

Juicing Tips for Beginners

It helps to know a few things before you get started on the juicing journey, as knowledge is power.

Experiment - First of all, you can juice pretty much any type of fruit or vegetables. Don't be scared to experiment. Just think "the more the merrier." As you walk through the supermarket, consider trying something you never have before.

Get a grocery list started - Get out your recipes and make a list of all the ingredients you will need. Planning makes it much easier to juice when you need to.

Prepare your vegetables and fruits the night before a morning juicing session. This means washing the produce, peeling them if needed, and storing them overnight in airtight containers.

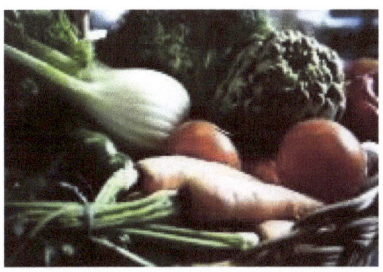

Nuts and Seeds - You should never juice nuts, grains or seeds, but instead grind and stir them into your ready-made juice. Adding nuts and seeds is a great way to boost the nutritional value of the juice and get many health benefits, but remember a little goes a long way.

Protein Powders - Protein powder can be added to juices when you drink them as a meal replacement so you get the protein you need.

Choose organic – Organic produce is more expensive, unless you buy from local farms when available, but you will ingest less pesticide and more nutrients.

Timing is everything when it comes to juicing. You don't want to be drinking your healthy fresh juice on a full stomach! If you do, your body just won't absorb all those lovely nutrients as well and some of them may even go to waste. A juice is best drank on an empty stomach. It's not going to fill you completely, but it will give your body a great chance to absorb all that goodness. Then, you can sit down to a meal an hour later.

Don't drink too quickly - this puts a LOT of pressure on your digestive enzymes that have to work extra hard to digest juice that is frank too fast. The best way to drink juice is to sit back and relax. Take care of your stomach and digestive tract because they are really sensitive.

Thoroughly wash your produce - This removes bacteria and some of the pesticide residue if you did not buy organic. This is especially important with leafy greens where dirt can be stuck in between the leaves.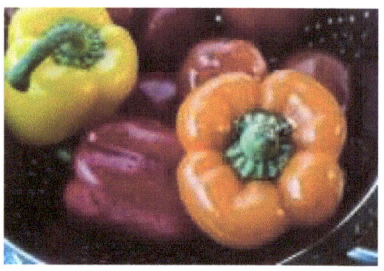

Line the pulp basket in the juicer - If your juicer has a pulp basket, you will need to line it with a plastic bag. This makes cleaning up the juicer afterward much easier.

Cut the produce so it fits - You can tear up the greens or cut up the larger vegetables so that it fits through the feeding chute of the juicer.

Read your juicer's user manual – This is very important because you will learn best practices for cutting produce, and also which speeds should be used for which fruits and vegetables. This will not only yield you the best juice, but will prevent breakage of the machine. For example, usually harder vegetables are best juiced on high, while softer vegetables, such as cabbage and spinach, are best juiced on a lower setting.

Rerun the pulp - In order to get the most nutrients out of the juice, take out the pulp, and run it through the juicer again to get more juice from the damp, left over pulp.

Clean the juicer right after use - You should do this right away so as to keep bacteria from building up inside the juicer. If it is dishwasher safe, you can put those parts in the dishwasher. Otherwise, you should scrub the juicer out with hot or warm water and a mild dish soap. Allow the juicer to dry on a drying mat rather than drying it out with a towel as this can get towel fibers in your next batch of juice.

Drink your juice while its fresh - The nutrients will go away if you keep the juice sitting too long and also remember that this is not store bought juice full of preservatives so it will not keep fresh as long. Put any leftover juice in a glass or BPA-free plastic airtight container in the refrigerator for no longer than 3 days.

Tips For Storing Juice

- If you are making a double batch, separate the batches and put the juice you are not drinking in the refrigerator right way.
- Fill the container to the top. You want to have as little space in the container as possible. If you have too much space, the oxygen in the container will begin to destroy the delicate micronutrients.
- If you want to freeze your juice, make sure you do so immediately after juicing, and for no longer than 7 to 10 days.

Eight Green Juice Recipes

How you prep and juice these ingredients will depend on your model of juicer, make sure to read the user manual and all instructions as different speed settings are used for different fruits and vegetables.

Green Energy Juice

It's easy to juice; simply push all the above ingredients into your juicer and go for it. It's incredibly energizing, and does more your for health, wellbeing and mental alertness than your usual cup of coffee. It's a fantastic way to start the day.

Ingredients:

- 5 Kale Leaves
- 3 Cups Spinach
- 1 Green Apple
- 1" Piece Of Ginger
- 1 Sprig Of Mint

Sweet Berry Green Juice

Here is a very simple green recipe where the sweet antioxidant rich berries blend perfectly with the nutrient dense kale.

How To:

1. Juice 5 Kale leaves

2. Blend 1 cup of any berries you like, strawberries, raspberries, etc. You can use a blender, a food processor or just mash the berries with a fork if time allows.

Add the berry puree to your kale juice, mix with a spoon, and enjoy!

Optional: For added zing, and to boost the nutrient content, juice ½ a lemon or lime with the kale, and/or juice a 1" piece of ginger.

Oh My Sweet Basil

Ingredients:

- 1 Handful Of Basil Leaves
- 1 Apple
- 1 Cucumber
- ¼ Lime
- 3 Spinach Leaves

Juice everything, starting with the basil leaves. Stir, top with a handful of ice cubes, and drink. It's so refreshing!

Spicy Green Juice

Okay, this one has a nice kick; as it includes Jalapeño that proves green juices can be really exciting and adventurous.

Ingredients:

- 1/2 Cup Of Fresh Pineapple
- 5 Kale Leaves
- ½ Piece Of Fresh Jalapeño
- 1 Cucumber

You could use a full jalapeño if you're feeling brave, but remember to warn your friends first!

Citrus Green Juice

If you can't handle the heat but still want a green juice that comes with a bit of a kick, try this citrus-inspired juice that proves green juicing can be tropical.

Ingredients:

- 1 Orange
- 2 Kale Leaves
- 3 Celery Stalks
- ½ Grapefruit
- ½ Cucumber
- ½ Lemon

Green Juice Cleanse

Here is one made with simple greens when you want to cleanse your body and get a big nutrition boost. This one is nice and simple and contains the classic dark leafy greens.

Ingredients:

- 4-5 Handfuls Of Spinach
- 3 Kale Leaves
- 2 Green Apples
- 3 Celery Stalks
- 1 Cucumber
- ½ Lemon

Liquid Broccoli Zinger

Ingredients:

- 1 Bunch Of Broccoli (Florets And Stalks)
- 2 Green Apples
- 1 Lime
- ½ Grapefruit
- 1/2 Small Zucchini
- Handful Of Spinach Or Romaine Lettuce Leaves
- 3 Stalks Of Celery

Green Honeymoon

Ingredients:

- 1 Cucumber
- 1 Apple
- ¼ Cup of Pineapple
- 4 Kale Leaves
- 3 Swiss Chard Leaves

A Word Of Caution

One pitfall is to avoid becoming so enamored with green juice that you forget about the other good stuff. You focus on kale and spinach, but you forget about beets and tomatoes. You buy lots of cabbages and broccoli, but you ignore the apples and carrots.

This is somewhat problematic because, although green vegetables are great for you, nutritionists and health experts all around the world will tell you that there is nothing better than a well-balanced diet - and this extends to a well-balanced diet of fruits and vegetables when juicing.

If you eat just certain kinds of vegetables, you'll be healthy. Sure. However, if you eat a wide variety of fruit and vegetables, you'll be even healthier.

SO, GET INTO GREEN JUICING BUT DON'T MAKE EVERY SINGLE JUICE GREEN. BE CREATIVE AND DYNAMIC; EXPERIMENT AND EXPLORE A VARIETY OF COLORFUL VEGETABLES TO ADD TO YOUR JUICE.

Conclusion

Your body needs the micronutrients found in fruit and vegetables, and juicing is a really great way of getting them. Furthermore, if you don't enjoy eating whole produce, juicing can help you get key nutrients that vegetables provide.

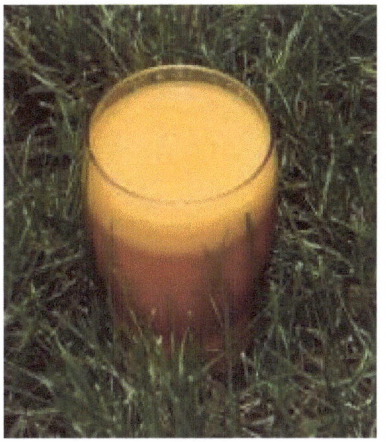

In fact, one large glass of juice is like eating 2 large salads without the fattening dressing.

You don't have to juice every single day, but it's great if you can make it a fundamental part of your daily routine.

Because most people who start juicing tend to really love it, it invariably becomes a crucial part of their daily routine. It becomes a habit that they don't ever want to lose.

There are just so many benefits...

- You feel more energized

- More alert

- Your immune system gets a boost

- Your bones are strengthened

- You stay hydrated

- Your skin looks better

- You supply your body with the nutrition it needs to fight disease

And you may lose some weight...

What More Could You Ask For?

Other Senior Health and Fitness Books by This Author

If you would like to read more about Senior Health and Fitness, here is a list of the <u>titles, CreateSpace links and descriptions:</u>

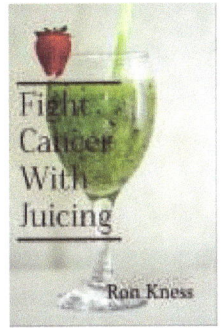

Fight Cancer With Juicing

https://www.createspace.com/6155567

Juicing is a healthy practice that has allowed millions of people to boost their nutrition. Juicing fruits and vegetables provides you important antioxidants, which scavenge for oxygen free radicals that can damage cellular structures, including DNA. When DNA is damaged, it can result in mutations that lead to cancer.

Well-balanced nutrition from a variety of healthy whole foods helps support and maintain on-going good health, and experts agree that nutrition plays a key role in preventing chronic and terminal illness.

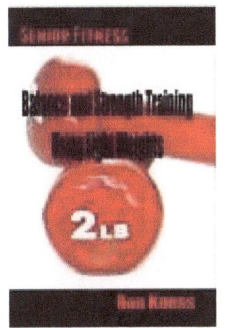

Senior Fitness – Balance and Strength Training Using Light Weights

https://www.createspace.com/6107842

As you age you notice that you are not as strong as before. Most of us simply chalk that up to the "natural" aging process. However, to fight the physical dangers of aging, strength is very important.

We are not talking about bodybuilding and packing on bulky muscles. What we mean is simply making your body stronger so that you don't become a statistic.

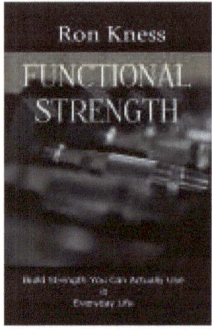

Functional Strength – Build Strength You Can Actually Use
https://www.createspace.com/6114822

Health and fitness fads come and go all the time but unfortunately not all of them are worth your time and effort. Some of them don't work, some of them are over-hyped and some of them are just plain dangerous.

But 'functional strength' is different. While functional strength is very much in vogue right now, it's not a 'fad' by any means. In fact, functional strength is the opposite of a fad and it's a step in the right direction for all of fitness.

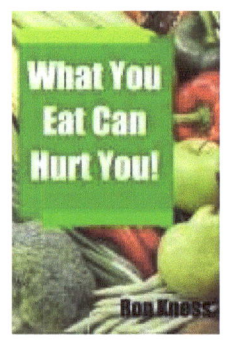

What You Eat Can Hurt You

https://www.createspace.com/4963196

Do you know that certain foods increase your risk for inflammation, disease and illness? It's true! And certain foods can help cure and heal you if you do get sick. Knowing which foods to eat and which ones to avoid empowers you to manage your own health.

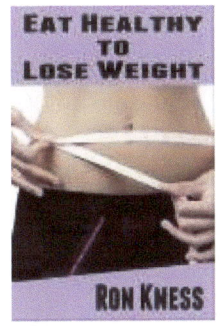

Eat Healthy to Lose Weight

https://www.createspace.com/4962939

As you read through our book, we show you which foods you should and should not be eating to reach your weight loss goal, along with discussing how to maintain your weight loss and stay within a few pounds of your goal weight. Banish the weight you keep gaining back each time by learning how to live a healthy lifestyle.

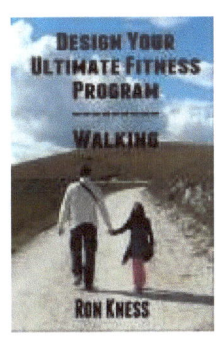

Design Your Ultimate Fitness Program - Walking

https://www.createspace.com/5252272

In my book Design Your Ultimate Fitness Program – Walking, we discuss the considerations that need to be made when designing a custom walking program, along with:

• Equipment needed
• Wearable technology you can use to track your walking
• And how to make walking more challenging

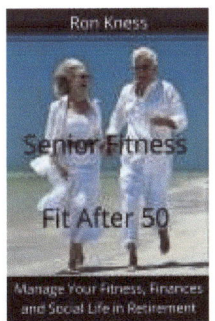

Senior Fitness – Fit After 50: Learn How to Manage Your Fitness, Finances and Social Life in Retirement

https://www.createspace.com/5474751

Inside you will discover answers to your most pressing questions:
• What do I need to know about downsizing my home?
• What are the best tips for staying healthy as you approach your 50's?
• When should I start planning for retirement?
• I am worried about being lonely once I retire, do others feel the same?
• Is it worthwhile to carry two homes during retirement?
And more…

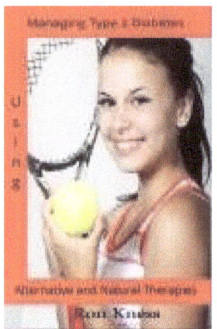

Managing Type 2 Diabetes Using Alternative And Natural Therapies

https://www.createspace.com/5401244

While Type 2 diabetes can be managed medically, there are many alternative natural and holistic methods of therapy and treatment that can further enhance quality of life and minimize the effects of this disease. In this book, I discuss 12 different types, including yoga, reflexology and acupuncture to name just three.

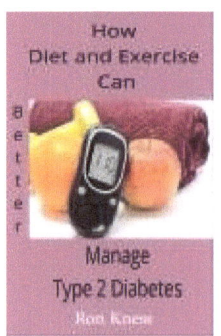

How Diet and Exercise Can Better Manage Type 2 Diabetes

https://www.createspace.com/5404845

Of the different types of diabetes, only Type 2 can be reversed. In my book How Diet and Exercise Can Better Manage Type 2 Diabetes,

we reveal the three things you can do to best manage your disease, including:
• Diet
• Exercise
• Weight management

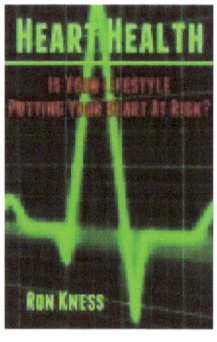

Heart Health: Is Your Lifestyle Putting Your Heart at Risk?

https://www.createspace.com/5464020

In my ebook Is Your Lifestyle Putting Your Heart At Risk? we discuss the six greatest risks to your heart and the lifestyle changes you can make to mitigate them.

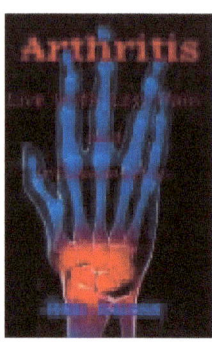

Arthritis – Live Wth Less Pain and Inflammation: Tips and Techniques You Can Use to Lessen the Pain and Inflammation

https://www.createspace.com/5457441

Discover Simple Tips & Information That Will Help Reduce The Painful Symptoms Of Arthritis!

You learn things like:
• Simple and effective information that will help you manage the pain and inflammation that comes along with arthritis, so that you can live an active, full life without debilitating pain.
• The different types of arthritis, their symptoms and how to alleviate their painful side effects.
• The pros and cons of over-the-counter arthritis medications, plus simple tips that will help you know how to choose the right supplements.
• Free, yet effective ways to get relief from arthritis pain and inflammation, so you don't have to suffer anymore.

the effects arthritis can have significant impact on your physical and mental well-being, but this books shows you how to overcome its painful symptoms and live life relatively pain free.

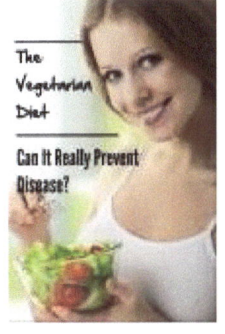

The Vegetarian Diet – Can It Really Prevent Disease?

https://www.createspace.com/5519874

Is a vegetarian diet right for you? Multiple studies have shown over and over that a vegetarian diet goes along way in preventing certain chronic diseases, such as:

• Heart Disease
• Cancer
• Diverticulitis
• Type 2 Diabetes
• Hypertension
• Obesity
• Kidney Failure

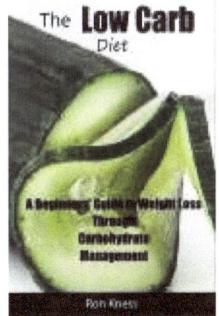

The Low Carb Diet: A Beginner's Guide to Weight Loss Through Carbohydrate Management

https://www.createspace.com/5416348

In my book "The Low-Carb Diet – A Beginners' Guide to Weight Loss Through Carbohydrate Management", I reveal a successful method of losing weight based in part on the amount and type of carbohydrates you consume.

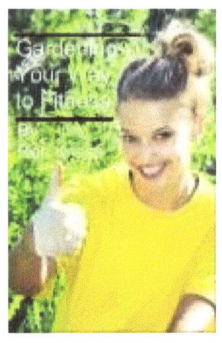

[Gardening Your Way to Fitness: The Fun Way to Get Fit and Provide Beauty and Healthful Bounty for Your Family](https://www.createspace.com/5459564)

https://www.createspace.com/5459564

The gym is a great place to stay fit during the colder seasons, but once the temperature turns warmer you want to spend more time outside. Plus, you'll have the benefit of fresh wholesome produce to enjoy by growing vegetables in your backyard garden.

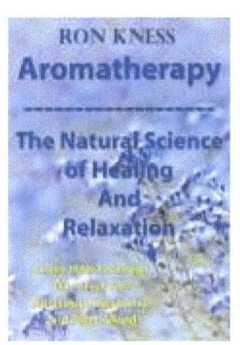

[Aromatherapy - The Science of Healing and Relaxation: Learn How Essential Oils Elicit The Relaxation Response And Alter Mood](https://www.createspace.com/5714434)

https://www.createspace.com/5714434

In my book Aromatherapy – The Science of Healing and Relaxation, we reveal the natural holistics methods you can use to heal the body from certain medical issues and to relive stress through relaxation. In particular we talk about:
• Aromatherapy - what it is and how it works
• Essential Oils – how the effects of certain aromas differs from others
• Recipes – how to make your own essential oil combinations

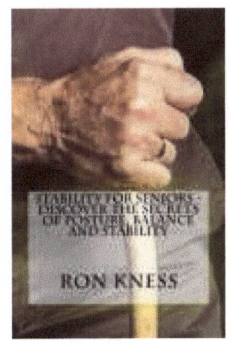

Stability for Seniors: Discover the Secrets of Posture, Balance and Stability

https://www.createspace.com/6096479

Many people sacrifice their health in pursuit of their career. They are so busy making a living that they neglect to make a life. The excuse that they do not have time to exercise is tossed about so frequently that they end up letting their health and fitness slide.

If you are not regularly active, you will have muscular atrophy over time. Your flexibility will decrease. Your core strength will diminish. As time progresses, you will be less limber and more rigid.

This is exactly how people age poorly. It's a process that has snowballed over time.

Only with regular exercise and a healthy diet can you have a body that is fit and has the ability to almost reverse aging.

If you have neglected your health for years and life seems to be a chore now because you can't get around without assistance, do not feel dejected.

You can remedy the situation. You can restore the strength, balance and stamina that you have lost. It is never too late to become what you might have been.

This guide will show you exactly what you need to do to restore your balance, strengthen your core and give you the ability to live life to its fullest. Read how …

About the Author

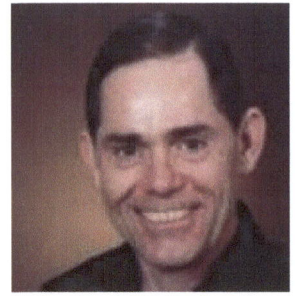

I grew up in Central Minnesota, where my parents own and operated a fishing resort. Once out of high school I tried a couple of semesters of college, only to quit halfway through the Spring term; I decided at that time that college wasn't for me.

Then I decided to follow my father's previous occupation as an auto mechanic. I graduated from a two-year of vocational training course and worked as a mechanic. While in vocational training, I decided to join the National Guard where I eventually ended up working full-time for 32 years.

So how does all of this relate to writing? In one of my leadership schools, the instructor, who was an English teacher at a juvenile detention center, presented writing to me in a whole new way - a way that started to develop my interest in working with words.

Fast forward about 40 years and I now have over 50 books listed on Amazon for Kindle and CreateSpace.

Today my wife and I live in Gold Canyon, AZ, where you'll find me happily sitting in my office typing away on my laptop as I work on my next book or ghostwriting project . . . that is if we are not traveling on a cruise ship - our new-found mode of travel.

If you like my book, please leave a review of it.